BREATHE DEEPLY, LIVE MODERATELY
& EAT LIGHTLY:
A Guide to Everyday Healthy Meals

ACKNOWLEDGEMENT

A special thank you to my mother, my rock, my inspiration, and the woman who taught me everything I know and everything I am. You instilled the importance of excellence at every level, and the significance of womanhood, health and education.

Thank you mommy! This one's for you!

Secondly, I would like to dedicate this to the spark of change— For the only way to truly survive is to stay informed, make better and healthier decisions, and to TAKE CARE OF ONE ANOTHER!

BREATHE DEEPLY, LIVE MODERATELY
& EAT LIGHTLY:
A Guide to Everyday Healthy Meals

Tyler Davis RN, MSN
Women's Gentle Care, Inc.

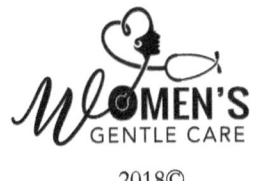

2018©

To contact the publisher or author, visit WOMENgentlecare.com

Tyler Davis, RN, MSN

Women's Gentle Care, Inc.

IBSN- 978-1-387-74406-0

Table of Contents

FOREWARD

The idea behind "Breathe Deeply, Live Moderately & Eat Lightly," is to ensure good health. By making meals packed with fruits and vegetables, you are guaranteed a moderately healthy lifestyle—not to mention these recipes contain the lowest amounts of sodium, fat, and sugar!

Eating the right amount of fruits and vegetables as part of a low fat, low sodium, high fiber diet may lower your risk of serious chronic conditions, such as obesity, heart disease and type 2 diabetes.

But, don't forget to be active! Yes, breathe deeply! Being physically active gives you more energy, which in return helps lowers stress factors. It also helps you maintain a healthy body weight–your body needs at least 30 minutes of moderate physical activity, whether walking, dancing, yoga, bike-riding, yard work, etc.

These recipe instructions were designed to help build your drive and keep you well-off along the greatest health path.

SALSA

Ingredients:
- 12 cups fresh chopped tomatoes
- ½ cup chopped jalapeño peppers
- 1 ½ cup chopped green bell peppers
- 4 large chopped yellow onions
- 1 tbsp. paprika
- 1 cup apple cider vinegar
- 1-12 oz. can of organic low-sodium tomato paste

How to Make it:

Mix chopped vegetables in a large bowel. In a separate bowel, mix apple cider vinegar, tomato paste, and seasonings together. Stir in apple cider vinegar mix into mixed vegetables. Enjoy!

*note you may cook in large sauce pan and let set, then serve cold, if desired.

VEGETABLE DIP

Ingredients:
- Low-Fat plain Greek yogurt
- 1 tbsp. Minced yellow onion
- 1 tsp. Apple cider vinegar
- 1 tsp. ginger (do not use if you are taking antiplatelet or anti-coagulant medication)
- 2 tbsp. Skim milk (stir in last)

How to Make it:

Mix and refrigerate. Serve the next day for best results.

DETOX SMOOTHIE

Ingredients:

- 3 cups frozen diced pineapple
- 3 cups fresh baby spinach
- 1 cup fresh peeled & diced banana
- 1 stick of celery
- 1 tbsp. chia seeds
- Juice from half a lime

How to Make it:

1. Blend.

BREAKFAST OATMEAL SMOOTHIE

Ingredients:

- ¼ cup old fashioned oats
- 1 fresh & peeled banana
- 1 cup unsweetened almond milk
- 1-2 tbsp. honey
- ½ tsp. ground cinnamon
- ½ tsp. vanilla extract
- pinch of nutmeg
- ¼ cup of raisins (optional)

How to Make it:

1. Add oats to blender, and pulse until finely grounded.
2. Add remaining ingredients and pulse until blended and smooth.
3. Serve immediately.

BERRY PROTEIN BREAKFAST SMOOTHIE

Ingredients:
- ½ cup of Silk Almond Dairy-free Vanilla Yogurt
- 1 scoop of protein powder of your choice (I use Nutiva Hemp protein powder)
- 1 cup frozen raspberries
- ¾ cup of unsweetened almond milk
- 2 tbsp. of raw berry honey

How to Make it:

1. Blend

Breathe Deeply, Live Moderately & Eat Lightly

SEVEN LAYER SALAD

Ingredients:
- 1 small head of lettuce, chopped into small pieces
- 1 cup of celery, chopped
- ½ cup green bell pepper, chopped
- 7 slices of turkey bacon, cut into pieces before frying, drain on paper towel
- 5 hard-boiled organic eggs, diced
- 1 cup non-fat Greek yogurt
- 1 cup sour cream

How to Make it:

1. Layer each of the above ingredients, in a dish of your choosing
2. Mix Greek yogurt and sour cream together, and spread over the top layer
3. Cover and refrigerate overnight

GARDEN SALAD

Ingredients:
- ½ head butter lettuce
- 1 box/bag serving of mixed spring greens
- 1 head organic cauliflower
- 1 head organic broccoli
- 1 pkg. Radishes
- 1 green bell pepper
- 2 large Persian cucumbers
- 1 yellow onion
- 1 tbsp. Extra virgin olive oil
- 1 tbsp. Raw honey
- 1 tbsp. Dijon mustard
- 2 tbsp. Apple Cider vinegar

How to Make it:

1. Chop vegetables into bite size pieces, then combine in a big salad bowl with lettuce and spring greens
2. In a separate bowl, mix together olive oil, raw honey, Dijon mustard, and apple cider vinegar. Once thoroughly mixed, stir into salad bowel
3. Refrigerate and serve chilled

BROCCOLI-ROMAINE SALAD

Ingredients:
- 1 ½ cup broccoli, chopped
- 1 cup celery, diced
- 1 cup green onions, chopped
- ½ cup red onions, chopped
- ½ cup green bell pepper, chopped
- 1 cup seedless red grapes, cut into halves
- 1 head of romaine lettuce, chopped
- 1 tbsp. Extra virgin Olive oil
- 1 tbsp. Sour cream
- 1 tsp. Red wine vinegar (any vinegar can work)

How to Make it:

1. Combine all fruit and vegetables in a large salad bowel
2. Mix together olive oil, sour cream, and vinegar to taste. Stir into salad bowl mixture
3. Refrigerate, and serve chilled

KALE-LEMON SALAD

Ingredients:
- 5 cups kale, chopped
- 1 avocado, diced
- ½ cup cooked quinoa
- ½ cup pomegranate
- ½ cup chopped pecans
- ¼ cup crumbled goat cheese
- ¼ cup extra virgin olive oil
- ¼ cup apple cider vinegar
- 3 tbsp. freshly squeezed Meyer lemon juice (sweeter flavor)
- zest from 1 Meyer lemon
- 1 tsp. Raw honey

How to Make it:

1. In a small bowl, mix together olive oil, apple cider vinegar, lemon juice, lemon zest and honey
2. In a large salad bowl, toss kale, avocado, quinoa, pomegranate, pecans and goat cheese
3. Stir in olive oil mixture
4. May add lemon wedges as garnish, if desired
5. Serve & enjoy

Breathe Deeply, Live Moderately & Eat Lightly

APPLE OATMEAL

Ingredients:
- 1 ¾ cup 100% apple juice
- 1 cup steal cut oats
- 1 granny-smith apple, cored and cut into bite sizes
- ½ tsp. ground cinnamon

How to Make it:

1. Combine all ingredients in a medium, microwave safe bowl
2. Cook in microwave for 2-3 minutes
3. Stir and let cool
4. Serve

FRESH FRUIT WAFFLES

Ingredients:
- 1 ¼ cup unsweetened almond milk
- 1 tsp. apple cider vinegar
- ¼ cup olive, canola or melted coconut oil
- ¼ cup agave nectar or maple syrup
- ½ cup gluten free rolled oats
- 1 ¾ cups gluten free flour blend
- 1 ½ baking powder
- 1 tsp. vanilla extract
- ½ tsp. cinnamon
- ½ tbsp. flax seed meal
- ¼ cup bananas, chopped

How to Make it:

1. Combine almond milk and vinegar in a small mixing bowl and let set for a few minutes to activate. Then add olive oil, agave nectar or maple syrup and whisk. Set aside
2. In a large mixing bowl, add dry ingredients and whisk until well combined.
3. Add wet ingredients to dry and mix well

4. Test batter for sweetness and flavor. Add vanilla extract, cinnamon, and flax seed meal
5. Let set for 5-10 minutes while your waffle iron preheats.
6. Once waffle iron is ready, generously coat with a non-stick spray and pour on about ½ cup of batter. Cook according to manufacturer instructions and then remove and place on a baking rack in a 200°F oven to keep warm
7. Do not stack and instead keep them in a single layer to ensure crispiness remains
8. Serve with banana toppings

BLUEBERRY CINNAMON FRENCH TOAST

Ingredients:

Blueberry Compote:
- 2 pints fresh blueberries
- ¼ cup agave
- ½ Meyer lemon juice, and zest from this lemon
- 1 tsp. ground cinnamon

Cinnamon French Toast:
- 1 loaf French bread
- 2 cups all purpose flour
- 2 cups almond
- 3 tbsp. maple syrup
- 2 tsp. pure vanilla extract
- 1 tsp. ground cinnamon
- 1 tsp. extra virgin olive oil

How to Make it:

Blueberry Compote:
1. In a small saucepot over low heat, combine blueberries, agave, lemon juice, lemon zest, and cinnamon
2. Let simmer for 10 minutes. Set aside

Cinnamon French Toast:
1. Slice the bread into ¾ thick slices
2. In a medium bowl whisk together flour, almond milk, maple syrup, vanilla extract, & cinnamon
3. Heat olive oil in large non-stick skillet over medium high heat. Submerge each slice of bread in the almond milk batter to coat, and then heat on skillet
4. Flip each French Toast, one by one, and let cook until lightly browned and crisp on both sides
5. Serve topped with the Blueberry Compote

SPINACH & TOMATO-EGG WHITE OMELET

Ingredients:
- ½ tsp. extra virgin olive oil
- 1 clove garlic, chopped
- 2 green onion, chopped
- 2 tbsp. low-fat cheddar cheese
- ¾ cup egg whites
- 1 large tomato, chopped
- ½ cup spinach, torn into pieces

How to Make it:

1. Prepare a medium non-stick pan with olive oil over medium heat. Pour in egg whites
2. When egg begins to set, approximately 1-2 minutes, spread evenly across the pan and reduce heat to low
3. Sprinkle the cheese, spinach, onions, garlic and tomato evenly over half of the omelet; fold the unfilled omelet half over the filing
4. Slide the cooked omelet on a plate and serve

CHICKEN BREAKFAST SKILLET

Ingredients:
- 6 oz. chicken sausage, casing removed
- 1 red bell pepper, chopped
- 1 small yellow onion, chopped
- 1 tbsp. of oil, if needed
- ½ lb. baby yellow potatoes
- 2 tbsp. Accent and ground pepper, mixed together
- 1 tbsp. of garlic, finely chopped
- ½ cup low-fat Monterey jack cheese
- 2 eggs
- 1 avocado, chopped
- 1 tbsp. fresh chives, finely chopped for garnish

How to Make it:

1. In a large, heavy bottomed skillet over medium heat, add the chicken sausage and break up with a wooden spoon
2. Cook until browned, about 10 minutes
3. Remove from the skillet and set aside
4. Add the pepper and onion to the skillet and cook in the chicken sausage grease until the onions are translucent, approximately 5 minutes
5. Remove the vegetables using a wooden spoon and set aside
6. If there is not enough grease left in the pan, add a tbsp. of oil.
7. Add in the potatoes and season with Accent and pepper
8. Cook, stirring every few minutes, until the potatoes are golden and crisp. Add the vegetables and chorizo back in with slotted spoon, making sure not to add too much of the grease back to the pan with them
9. Continue to cook 5-10 minutes, or until the potatoes are tender and cooked through
10. Add in the cheese and stir
11. Make two holes in the potato mixture and crack an egg into each well, and cook to your liking
12. Add avocado and chives
13. Serve

BREAKFAST POTATOES

Ingredients:
- 1 lb. red potatoes, scrubbed clean & dried
- 3-4 tbsp. extra virgin olive oil
- 1 tsp. Accent
- ½ tsp. garlic powder
- ½ tsp. ground black pepper

How to Make it:

1. Heat skillet to medium heat
2. Place the potatoes in the microwave for 4-6 minutes, flipping halfway through
3. Cut cooked potatoes into bite sized pieces, and olive oil on skillet. Place potatoes, one by one
4. After about 4 minutes use a fork to tip the potato over onto its other side to brown evenly
5. After 3-4 minutes, flip the potatoes on their backsides and season with Accent, pepper, and garlic powder. Cook for another 2-4 minutes until crispy and golden brown on all sides
6. Serve

CHICKEN WITH CUCUMBER SAUCE

Ingredients:
- 1 boneless organic chicken breast
- Flat bread
- ¼ plain non-fat Greek yogurt
- 1 tbsp. Cayenne pepper
- 1 tbsp. Garlic powder
- 1 tbsp. Onion powder
- ¼ cup of lime juice
- ½ tbsp. Accent seasoning
- Raw vegetables of your choice, including 4 Persian Cucumbers

- Mint leaves

How to Make it:

1. Mix yogurt and seasoning, then cut chicken into bite size
2. Let marinate
3. Mix ½ cup Greek yogurt, ¼ cucumber, mint leaves, Accent, cayenne pepper & black pepper, and refrigerate.
4. Put chicken on skewers & bake.
5. Top chicken with lime juice & raw veggies and spread cucumber sauce on top.

<u>CHICKEN QUESADILLAS</u>

Ingredients:
- 1 boneless organic chicken breast
- ½ bell pepper; chopped
- ½ onion; chopped
- 1 zucchini; chopped
- 1 garlic; chopped
- 1 tbsp. black pepper
- 1 tbsp. garlic powder
- 1 tbsp. onion powder
- 3 tbsp. cheddar cheese
- 4 whole grain flat tortillas

How to Make it:

1. Boil chicken on medium heat until it shreds
2. Sautee veggies in ½ tbsp. coconut oil until fragrant
3. Add chicken, and season with garlic powder, onion powder and black pepper
4. In a separate skillet or grill, cook tortillas and add chicken mixture and top with cheese
5. Half tortilla & press down gently to adhere together
6. Serve & enjoy

TURKEY MEAT BALLS

Ingredients:
- 2 garlic cloves, chopped
- 1 jalapeno halved & seeded, chopped
- 1 pound lean ground turkey
- 1 large egg lightly beaten
- 1 tbsp. almond milk
- ¼ cup flour, for dusting
- 1 small can of tomato paste
- 1 tbsp. garlic powder
- 1 tbsp. onion powder
- 1 tbsp. black pepper
- ½ tsp. oregano
- 1 tbsp. parsley
- 2 tbsp. olive oil

How to Make it:

1. Mix chopped vegetables, and add to large bowl & stir in turkey, egg, and milk.
2. Roll mixture into 15-20 balls
3. Dust balls with flour
4. Add oregano, remaining garlic & half jalapeno (chopped) then make smooth.
5. Heat olive oil, add ball & cook for 5-6 min.
6. Add tomato sauce to skillet for 2 min.
7. Sprinkle Parsley
8. Serve

LOW CARB BBQ CHICKEN PIZZA

Ingredients:
- Low Carb Whole Wheat Tortilla Wrap—gluten free or vegan options may be substituted
- Reduced sodium BBQ
- Spinach
- Boneless Organic Chicken Breast

- Assorted Bell Peppers
- Chopped Yellow and Green Onions
- Chopped Garlic Cloves
- Broccolini
- Mozzarella Cheese

How to Make it:

1. Preheat oven to 350°F
2. Toast wrap in oven for 5 minutes
3. Boil chicken on medium heat until it shreds
4. Sautee spinach, shredded chicken, bell peppers, broccolini, chopped garlic cloves & onion
5. Spread BBQ sauce of your choice to the toasted wrap, sprinkle cheese, and add sautéed ingredients
6. Bake pizza wrap with ingredients for 7-10 minutes, if desired, then serve

PARMESAN GARLIC CHICKEN WINGS

Ingredients:
- 2lbs party chicken wings
- 1 tsp. dried oregano
- 1 tsp. dried rosemary
- ½ tsp. ground cumin
- ½ tsp. Accent
- 1 tsp. garlic powder
- 1 tsp. onion powder
- 2 tbsp. olive oil
- 6 fresh basil leaves, chopped
- 2 cloves garlic, chopped
- ¼ cup grated parmesan cheese
- 1 tsp. lemon zest

How to Make it:

1. Rinse and clean the chicken wings. Pat dry with paper towels, set aside in big bowl
2. Preheat oven to 425°F. Add the oregano, rosemary, cumin, Accent, garlic powder and onion powder to the clean chicken wings. Toss to combine well so each chicken wing is nicely coated with seasoning and spices.
3. Transfer the chicken wings on a baking sheet and bake for about 25-30 minutes, or until the chicken wings turn to a nice brown color.
4. In a separate bowel, mix the olive oil, basil, garlic, lemon zest and parmesan cheese together
5. Transfer the chicken wings out of the oven and toss them with the Parmesan mixture.
6. Serve

CHICKEN FAJITA QUESADILLAS

Ingredients:
- 3 tbsp. olive oil
- 2 tbsp. ground cumin
- 2 tbsp. ground turmeric
- 3 boneless chicken breasts
- 1 red bell pepper
- 1 green bell pepper
- 1 yellow onions
- ½ cup low-fat cheddar cheese
- 8 tortillas
- 1 avocado

How to Make it:

1. Clean and chop up the onion and bell peppers into long strips.
2. Clean and slice the chicken breasts into long strips and place in a separate bowl.
3. Add the cumin and turmeric to the chicken breast and mix well

4. In a large skillet, heat the first tbsp. of olive oil and add the chicken to it
5. Cook the chicken for 5 -10 minutes until it's fully cooked and no longer pink, and it's slightly charred, but not burned
6. Remove chicken from skillet, and wipe the skillet clean
7. Add the second tbsp. of olive oil to the skillet and heat
8. Add the onion and cook for a couple minutes until its slightly translucent
9. Add the peppers and the cumin & turmeric mix
10. Cook for a couple more minutes so the peppers cook slightly
11. Add the chicken to the skillet, mix with peppers and onions, and cook
12. In a separate clean skillet, add the third tbsp. of olive oil
13. Add a tortilla. Add a little bit of the chicken and onion mixture to half of the tortilla, and cheese, depending on how you like it
14. Add another tortilla on top and pat it down until flat
15. Flip it over and cook on the other side until the other side is nice and golden
16. Remove from skillet and cut into quarters
17. Repeat these steps with the remaining tortillas
18. Halve and slice Avocado
19. Serve with Avocado slices

FIRE ROASTED TOMATO PASTA

Ingredients:
-   9 oz. canned in water chopped tomatoes
-   1 lb. whole wheat penne pasta
-   6 oz. fresh spinach
-   10 oz. fresh cherry tomatoes
-   4 garlic cloves, chopped
-   ¼ cup low-fat parmesan cheese, grated
-   ¼ cup fresh parsley
-   ½ tsp. Accent
-   1 tbsp. olive oil

How to Make it:

1. Boil pasta according to package instructions
2. In a large non-stick skillet, over medium to high heat, heat the oil
3. Add the garlic and cook for 1 minute, just until fragrant. Add the chopped cherry tomatoes and Accent, and sauté
4. Stir in the in water canned tomatoes. Turn the heat off and add the fresh spinach
5. Add the cooked pasta, fresh parsley and parmesan cheese to the skillet and mix the ingredients through
6. Serve

KALE AND SPINACH ROTINI PESTO PASTA

Ingredients:
- 16 oz. Rotini pasta, any of choice
- 4 oz. fresh spinach
- 4 oz. fresh baby kale
- 4 oz. frozen peas
- 4 oz. pesto sauce
- ½ tsp. Accent

How to Make it:

1. Cook pasta according to package instruction, about 8-10mins
2. Place peas in a microwave safe dish and microwave for 4 minutes, depending on the power of the microwave, until they are warm
3. Transfer pasta to a big skillet pan and add the remaining ingredients
4. Stir until thoroughly mixed
5. Serve

VEGGIE CHILI

Ingredients:

- 15 chopped cherry tomatoes
- ½ bag of kidney beans
- ½ bag of butter beans
- ½ red bell pepper, chopped
- ½ green bell pepper, chopped
- ½ white onion, chopped
- 2 garlic cloves, chopped
- 16 oz. vegetable stock
- 3 oz. red wine
- 2 tsp. cumin
- 4 tsp. chili powder
- 2 tsp. paprika
- 1 tsp. plain white flour
- ½ tsp. black pepper
- ½ tsp. Accent
- ½ tsp. dried basil
- 2 tbsp. olive oil

How to Make it:

1. Soak beans the day before for best results. Cook beans according to package instructions
2. Mix together all of the spices, seasoning, herbs, flour and sugar in a small bowl. (This is what will pack all of the punch in your chili). Make sure it is well mixed and put it to the side
3. Drain water from beans, and add vegetable stock. Stir well on low heat.
4. Whilst your beans and vegetable stock is cooking, stir in spice mixture.
5. In a separate skillet, pour olive oil, put on a medium heat and sauté the pepper, garlic, and onion for 3-4 minutes or until the onions become translucent. Then add the vegetables to the pot with the beans, followed by the red wine and bring the chili to the boil. Stir well.

6. Reduce the heat and leave your chili for as long as you've got.
7. Serve to taste

CROCK POT KUNG PAO CHICKEN

Ingredients:
- 2 lbs. Boneless chicken breast, cut into 1" cubes
- 1 tsp. Accent
- 1 tsp. black pepper
- 1 tbsp. onion powder
- 2 tbsp. olive oil
- ½ cup low sodium chicken broth
- ¼ cup balsamic vinegar
- 2 tbsp. organic coconut aminos sauce
- 6-10 dried red chili peppers, split & seeds removed (adjust according to desired heat level)
  - 1 orange bell pepper, chopped
  - 1 yellow bell pepper, chopped
  - ½ medium white onion, chopped
  - 4 cloves garlic, minced
  - 1 tsp. fresh ginger, minced
  - 2 tbsp. cornstarch
  - Peanuts or cashews, to top (optional)
  - Green onion, to garnish

How to Make it:

1. Heat oil in a skillet over medium-high heat. Season the chicken breast with Accent, black pepper, and onion powder. Sauté until browned on all sides. Add chicken to the crock-pot
2. In the crock-pot, add in the chicken broth, balsamic vinegar, sugar, and coconut aminos sauce. Give the pot a light stir. Then, add in the chili peppers, bell peppers, onion, garlic, and ginger. Continue to stir. Cover and cook on low heat for 4 hours

3. Around the 3 hour and 30 minute mark, combine equal parts water and cornstarch in a small bowl, mix until smooth. Add to the crock-pot and mix well.
4. Continue to cook for another 30 minutes, or until sauce has thickened
5. While you wait for the sauce to thicken, cut the green onions for garnishing
6. Serve topped with garnish

** You may enjoy this meal over brown rice, if desired**

VEGGIE LEMON PESTO

Ingredients:
- 8 oz. whole wheat penne
- 2 cups baby broccoli
- 1 cup cherry tomatoes, chopped
- 1 tsp. garlic cloves, minced
- ¼ cup low-sodium pesto
- ¼ cup low-fat feta cheese
- ¼ cup lemon juice
- 1 tbsp. fresh basil, chopped

How to Make it:

1. Cook the penne according to package directions. Add the baby broccoli to the pot of boiling water for the last 1-2 minutes of cooking. It should turn bright green
2. Drain and return penne and broccoli contents to the pan over medium high heat
3. Add the tomatoes and garlic to the pan. Sauté until fragrant
4. Add pesto, the feta cheese, and the lemon juice to the pan until well combined. Remove from heat and add the basil
5. Serve

BBQ CHICKEN PARTY WINGS

Ingredients:
- 2 tsp. paprika
- 2 tsp. Accent
- ½ tsp. black pepper
- 2 tsp. garlic powder
- ½ tsp. cayenne pepper
- 1 tsp. cumin
- 1 tsp. brown sugar
- 1 12 pack of party wings
- ¼ cup of G Hughes Smokehouse sugar free BBQ sauce

How to Make it:

1. Combine the spices in a small bowl.
2. Rub the mixture over clean, dry chicken pieces and leave to marinate (anywhere from 30 minutes to overnight)
3. Heat a large pan over medium high heat and brown the seasoned chicken well on both sides.
4. Heat the oven to 375°F, and place the chicken on a cookie sheet
5. Lightly glaze with BBQ sauce then transfer to the oven
6. Bake until the chicken is done, approximately 30-45 minutes, brushing with BBQ sauce every 10 minutes until the ¼ cup is empty
7. Remove from oven and let rest at least 5 minutes to cool
8. Serve

VEGGIE FLATBREAD

Ingredients:
- 4 pita breads of naan
- 1 cup crumbled low-fat feta cheese
- 1 cup artichokes, chopped
- 1 cup cherry tomatoes, chopped
- 3 green onions, chopped
- ¼ cup parsley, chopped
- 1 tsp. olive oil

- 1 tbsp. black pepper
- 1 tsp. Accent

How to Make it:

1. Preheat oven to 400°F.
2. Place pita breads in single layer on baking sheet
3. In a skillet sauté artichoke and tomatoes with olive oil, on low heat for 10 mins
4. Top pita breads with sautéed artichokes and tomatoes, and top with cheese
5. Bake for 10 to 12 mins or until heated through
6. Garnish with onions and parsley and season with black pepper and Accent

SHRIMP AND SNOW PEAS STIR FRY WITH CHILI, MISO & TOMATO

Ingredients:
- ½ tbsp. miso paste
- 2 tbsp. tomato paste
- 4 tbsp. tepid water
- 2 tsp. extra virgin olive oil
- pinch of Accent
- 200g snow peas, trimmed & washed
- 1 long red chili, deseeded & chopped
- 2 scallion onions, sliced
- 400g peeled shrimps
- ½ tsp. ground white pepper
- 2 drops of sesame oil

How to Make it:

1. In a small bowl, whisk miso paste, tomato paste, and 4 tbsp. of tepid water until well combined with a fork. Set aside

2. In a large pan, add olive oil. When the oil is hot, add snow peas with a pinch of Accent. Sauté until they turned bright green, slightly soft but with a bit of crunch. Transfer to a plate and keep warm
3. In the same pan, add the chopped chili and the white section of the sliced scallion onions
4. When the chili and onions become fragrant, add shrimp and season with white pepper. Sauté until they just turned opaque
5. Add the miso-tomato paste mixture to the shrimp and cook until the sauce is heated through
6. Add the drops of sesame oil before removing the stir fry from the heat
7. Serve

ROSEMARY BALSAMIC BABY POTATOES & BRUSSELS
Ingredients:
- 9200g Brussels sprouts
- 440g baby potatoes
- 2 tbsp. balsamic vinegar
- 1 tbsp. extra virgin olive oil
- 1 tsp. dried rosemary
- 1 tsp. black pepper
- 1 tsp. Accent

How to Make it:

1. Preheat oven to 450°F
2. Cut off the ends of the Brussels sprouts and cut them in half. Cut the baby potatoes in half. Wash the Brussels sprouts and potatoes and put in a large bowl
3. Drizzle the olive oil and balsamic vinegar on the potatoes and Brussels sprouts. Season with Accent and pepper, then add rosemary. Toss well so seasoning is evenly distributed
4. Place potatoes and Brussels sprouts on a baking sheet and bake for about 30-40 minutes or until golden

CHICKEN PASTA WITH CREAMY CAULIFLOWER SAUCE

Ingredients:

- 2 tbsp. extra virgin olive oil
- 3 large garlic cloves, minced
- 3-4 oz. Fat-free sun-dried tomatoes
- 1 lb. Organic boneless chicken breast, thinly sliced
- ¼ tsp. Accent
- 1 ½ tsp. paprika, divided
- 4 cups spinach
- 1 cup cauliflower sauce
- 1 cup reserved cooked pasta water
- 1 tbsp. fresh basil
- ½ tsp. crushed red pepper
- 8 oz. fettuccine pasta

How to Make it:

1. Chop sun-dried tomatoes into bites sizes.
2. Lightly cover chicken breast in about ½ tsp. of paprika, for color
3. In a large pan, heat olive oil on medium-high heat, and sauté garlic, chopped sun-dried tomatoes and thinly sliced chicken breast for 2-3 minutes until chicken is cooked through, turning it over a couple of times. Sprinkle the Accent over the chicken and a little more paprika while cooking
4. Remove pan from heat. Immediately add fresh spinach, cover the skillet with the lid, and let everything rest off heat, until spinach wilts
5. Cook pasta according to package instructions. Reserve some cooked pasta water- about 1 cup
6. Drain and rise the pasta with cold water
7. Add 1 cup cauliflower sauce and ¼ cup reserved cooked pasta water to the chicken and sun-dried tomatoes. Add basil, 1 tsp. paprika, and crushed red pepper. Mix the sauce well

8. Stir in cooked pasta to the skillet with the creamy sauce. The sauce should not be too thick, add more water for a more creamy consistency
9. Serve

GREEK YOGURT MASHED POTATOES

Ingredients:
- 1 lb. russet potatoes, peeled and cut
- 4 tbsp. extra virgin olive oil
- ¼ cup Greek yogurt
- ¼ cup boiling water from the pan with cooked potatoes
- ¼ tsp. Accent
- 4 green onions, finely chopped

How to Make it:

1. Bring a large pot of water to boil. Add potatoes (peeled and cut). Cook for about 30 minutes until potatoes are fork tender. Remove from heat
2. Using a deep slotted spoon, move the potatoes from the pan with hot water into a large bowl. Reserve some of the cooked potato water
3. Using a potato masher, mash them slightly. Then, stir in olive oil, continuing to mash. Add ¼ cup of hot water from boiling the potatoes to the mashed potatoes, continuing to mash. Add Greek yogurt while continuing to mash. Season with Accent
4. Garnish with finely chopped green onions
5. Serve

ROASTED SHRIMP SCAMPI

Ingredients:
- 8 oz. shelled and deveined large sized shrimp
- 3 cloves garlic, minced
- 1 ½ tbsp. extra virgin olive oil
- 1 tbsp. white wine
- ½ tbsp. lemon juice

- 1 tbsp. chopped parsley leaves
- 3 dashes ground black pepper
- ½ tsp. red pepper flakes
- Lemon wedges, for serving

How to Make it:

1. Preheat the oven to 550°F for broiling.
2. Rinse the shrimp and pat dry with paper towels. In a baking dish, combine the shrimp with the rest of the ingredients, and stir well to combine
3. Transfer the baking dish to the oven and broil for 4-5 minutes, in the middle rack. Remove dish from the oven once cooked thoroughly
4. Serve immediately with some lemon wedges

** pairs well over pasta or rice

PARMESAN ZUCCHINI & GARLIC PASTA

Ingredients:
- 2 tbsp. extra virgin olive oil
- 4 small zucchinis, sliced
- 4 garlic cloves, minced
- 8 oz. Whole wheat spaghetti
- 1 tsp. black pepper
- 1 tsp. Accent
- 1 cup freshly shredded Parmesan cheese

How to Make it:

1. Heat olive oil in a large skillet on medium-high heat. Add sliced zucchini and minced garlic, and sauté for about 5-7 minutes, occasionally stirring, until zucchini softens and browns a bit, uncovered
2. Midway through cooking, season with Accent

3. Cook pasta according to pasta instructions. Drain and rise with cold water. On low heat, add cooked pasta into the skillet with zucchini and garlic
4. Add freshly shredded Parmesan cheese into the skillet and stir pasta on low heat to melt the cheese
5. Serve

BAKED GARLIC AND GINGER CHICKEN DRUMSTICKS

Ingredients:
- 12 chicken drumsticks
- 8 cloves garlic, minced
- 1 inch piece of ginger root, minced
- ½ cup fresh parsley, chopped
- ¼ cup
- ¼ cup extra virgin olive oil
- 1 tsp. Accent
- 1 tsp. black pepper
- 1 tsp. garlic powder
- 3 tbsp. organic coconut aminos

How to Make it:

1. Add all ingredients, not including drumsticks, to a blender and pulse until garlic and ginger are a paste and the mixture softens
2. Place the drumsticks in a large Ziploc bag and pour the blended mixture over the chicken. Close the bad and place in fridge to marinade for about 20 minutes. Could be marinated overnight, if desired
3. Preheat oven to 375°F
4. Place the chicken and all of the marinade in a baking pan. Bake for about 45 minutes or until chicken is cooked thoroughly and browned
5. Take dish out, and let sit for 5 minutes
6. Serve

CHICKEN, CORN AND SWEET POTATO CHOWDER

Ingredients:

- 1 lb. boneless, skinless chicken thighs, trimmed & cut into bite size pieces
- 1 tsp. Accent
- 1 tsp. freshly ground black pepper
- 2 tbsp. coconut oil
- 1 medium yellow onion, minced
- 3 celery sticks, minced
- 2 medium sweet potatoes cut into ½ inch cubes
- 3 tbsp. unbleached all purpose flour
- 1 tsp. thyme leaves
- 4 cups low sodium chicken broth
- 2 corn on the cobs, kernels removed
- 1 cup fat-free half & half
- 2 tbsp. chives, minced
- 2 tbsp. fresh parsley, chopped
- 1 tsp. fresh lemon juice

How to Make it:

1. Place a large saucepan over medium high heat and add 1 tsp. coconut oil
2. Season chicken generously on all sides with Accent & pepper. Working in batches, add chicken to the pan and cook, stirring occasionally until chicken is well browned on all sides, approximately 5-6 minutes
3. Transfer chicken to a medium bowl, set aside
4. Reduce heat to medium and add 1 tsp. to the pan. Once melted add the onions, celery, & sweet potatoes and cook until soft, approximately 3-4 minutes. Stir in flour and cook for 2-3 minutes to make a roux
5. Whisk in broth & corn, and stir until well combined. Simmer, stirring occasionally until mixture thickens and the sweet potatoes are tender for 6 minutes

6. Return the chicken to the pan and simmer until the chicken is cooked through, approximately 2 minutes. Whisk in half & half and chopped herbs, and add lemon juice to taste
7. Serve

ORAGNE-POMEGRANTE SALMON

Ingredients:
- 1 ½ wild Salmon fillet, cut into strips
- 2 tbsp. extra virgin olive oil
- 1 tsp. Accent
- 1 tsp. black pepper
- 1 tsp. garlic powder
- 1 tsp. onion powder
- 2 large ripe oranges, peeled and cut
- 3 cups baby arugula
- ¼ cup pomegranate seeds
- 1 tbsp. shallot, minced
- 1 tsp. lemon juice

How to Make it:

1. Season salmon generously on all sides with Accent, black pepper, garlic powder and onion powder. Set Aside
2. Add 1 tbsp. olive oil to a large nonstick pan over medium to high heat. Add salmon, and sear until crispy, approximately 4 minutes. Turn fish over, and cook for 3 more minutes
3. In a separate bowel, toss arugula, oranges and pomegranate seeds with 1 tbsp. olive oil.
4. Once salmon is very soft and pink, transfer on top of arugula mixture and drizzle lemon juice over
5. Serve

Breathe Deeply, Live Moderately & Eat Lightly

CINNAMON ROLLS

Ingredients:

- 1 packet yeast (instant)
- 1 cup almond milk
- 3 tbsp. & ¼ cup extra virgin olive oil, divided
- ¼ cup & 1 tbsp. sugar, divided
- 3 cups all purpose flour, divided
- ¼ tsp. salt substitute
- 1/3 cup Splenda sugar
- 1/3 cup light brown sugar
- 2 tbsp. cinnamon

How to Make it:

1. In microwave safe bowl, heat milk & ¼ cup olive oil at 30 minute increments until lukewarm
2. In separate bowl whisk 3 cups flour, Splenda, and salt substitute. Stir in yeast & milk mixture. Beat dough for 5 minutes on low speed, cover the bowl with a damp paper towel and let sit for 10 minutes
3. In another separate bowel, whisk 3 tbsp. olive oil, cinnamon, brown sugar and sugar together—this will be your filling
4. On a lightly floured surface, roll out the dough to thin rectangles. Brush with the cinnamon filling mixture, and cut into rectangles
5. Roll dough into circles
6. Place damp towel and set aside for 25min
7. When rolls have risen place in oven 350°F for 15-20 min
8. Serve

PEACH CRUMBLE

Ingredients:
- 4 cans juice packed peach slices, drained
- 2 tbsp. cornstarch
- 1 tsp. vanilla extract
- 1 ¼ ground cinnamon

- 2/3 cup old-fashioned oats
- ¼ cup brown sugar
- 1/3 cup all purpose flout
- 1 ½ tbsp. coconut oil

How to Make it:

1. Preheat oven to 400°F
2. Pour peaches into a non-stick pie pan
3. In a small bowl, stir in cornstarch, vanilla, and 1 tsp. cinnamon. Pour this mixture over the peaches
4. In a large bowl, mix remaining cinnamon, oats, brown sugar, flour and coconut oil. Sprinkle this mixture over peaches
5. Bake for 20-25 minutes
6. Serve

LEMON POUND CAKE

Ingredients:

- 1 ½ cups all purpose flour
- 2 tsp. baking powder
- ¼ tsp. salt substitute
- ¾ cup sugar in the raw, or Splenda sugar
- 1 Meyer lemon zest
- 1 ½ cup low-fat Greek yogurt
- ¼ cup almond milk
- ¼ cup extra virgin olive oil
- ½ tsp. vanilla extract
- 3 large eggs, use egg whites for 2 of them

How to Make it:

1. Preheat the oven to 350°F
2. Coat pan with baking spray
3. In a medium bowl, whisk together flour, baking powder and salt substitute

4. In a separate bowl, mix together the sugar and lemon zest. Add the Greek yogurt, milk, olive oil, vanilla, egg whites and whole egg and whisk until well blended
5. Combine the flour mixture and the egg mixture, and transfer to the prepared pan
6. Bake approximately 50 minutes
7. Take out of oven, let cool to room temperature
8. Serve

Breathe Deeply, Live Moderately & Eat Lightly

AFTERWORD

I am so happy to take this journey with you towards achieving a healthier lifestyle. I hope this new-start to a new you, will keep you motivated to do more!

The body needs a variety of the following 5 nutrients - protein, carbohydrate, fat, vitamins and minerals – And each recipe was designed with this in mind. Furthermore, by engaging in the choice of healthier food choices, we are able to combat excessive weight gain, or obesity. In doing so, the risks of chronic health problems like type 2 diabetes, heart disease, high blood pressure, is greatly minimized.

It is imperative to eat healthy and eat right in order to stay healthy!!!

Follow Women's Gentle Care, Inc. on Instagram @Womengentlecare_, visit our website WOMENgentlecare.com, and support our movement!

DON'T FORGET TO . . .
BREATHE DEEPLY, LIVE MODERATELY
& EAT LIGHTLY